A DIET DEDICATED TO ATHLETES

Michael H. Atkins

Copyright © 2022 by Michael H. Atkins

All rights reserved.

No portion of this book may be reproduced in any form without written permission from the publisher or author, except as permitted by U.S. copyright law.

Contents

1. INTRODUCTION 1

2. THE PROBLEM OF FOOD INTOLERANCE 7

3. How healthy is your gut? 11

4. UNDERSTANDING FOOD INTOLERANCES 15

5. Athlete's or food intolerance 25

6. When you want to perform well, eat well. 31

7. FIXING YOUR DIET 45

Chapter One

INTRODUCTION

To provide the necessary vitamins and minerals for the performance of exercise, a well-balanced diet must include various foods: fruits, vegetables, meats, fish, and dairy products. While most studies have shown that consuming less fat will improve the health of those who already are in good health, those who are in poor health may benefit as well by reducing fat. In addition, the recommended diet is composed of foods that are prepared from scratch.

I know it is wrong to cheat on my diet. Instead, I have been eating a clean diet. I have increased fiber intake to help with the feeling of water retention before a race. Sugar has been replaced with healthy carbs that fuel my body with fuel. However, I have not been feeling well. I have been bloating, experiencing a feeling of water retention, experiencing more lethargy, and experiencing shortness of breath.

2   A DIET DEDICATED TO ATHLETES

Since race day came along, I had been racing too much and was doing a diet heavy on gluten-containing foods. Then, I started to notice that wheat was having an effect. Maybe it was my body's reaction to consuming too much of it for a while. So, I cut out wheat and the effects were gone. I think because I was not overly strict and my body was used to gluten-free eating, I felt fine — although I wasn't sure if there was a real reason to go gluten free or if it was just because it was easier.

As I began to investigate the impact of food on my body, I began to strictly avoid inflammation-causing foods but I also discovered that I was sensitive to specific foods. I eliminated gluten, grains, and foods with milk products (especially heavy cream), and began focusing more heavily on proteins such as red meat, fish, poultry, and dairy. I also ate more vegetables and fruits. The headaches I had endured for years were improved, along with the brain fog. I felt physically and mentally strong when I ate the right foods. I didn't miss eating grains and I discovered that I was less hungry in general. I focused more on proteins such as red meat, fish, poultry, and dairy, and included plenty of healthy fats along with abundant vegetables and fruits.

Back in the days when I was a kid, my headaches started at the age of 11. They were frequent, but they never bothered me much. Whenever I suffered from one, no matter how bad it was, it would just subside after a few hours. I assumed it was normal for people to have bad headaches.

Iron, the mineral that is vital to blood formation and oxygen carriage, is responsible for much of the body's function, from keeping bones healthy to creating and transporting energy.

I have found that eating healthier foods is the best approach to making and maintaining good health in my own life. I have also found that some people are able to gain weight and not feel great about it, while others can lose weight and feel great about it. However, there is evidence of the benefits of a low-fat diet for reducing chronic symptoms in people with endometriosis and fibromyalgia.

You can control and change the diet that supports your running performance and improves your stamina. Your diet, including your protein intake, will directly affect your running performance, as well as contribute to overall body health and well-being. You must examine the diet that is best for you and your long-term goals.

Athletes often have trouble with their diets. They need to make sure that their healthy meal plans provide protein for muscle growth and support a lean figure. However, they often find it difficult to identify which of his sports drinks or energy bars should they be consuming, and even harder to understand how much and what kind of nutritional supplements to take.

4   A DIET DEDICATED TO ATHLETES

For better or worse, we are all encouraged to eat a wide variety of foods. We are told that there is no single diet that will work for everyone. There are too many products, many of which are harmful. We are told to eat foods that are beneficial. We are told that every food has the potential to be good for our bodies.

Health is affected by the choices and actions we make every day, especially when it comes to food.

The Athlete's Fix is a simple and effective guide to help you find your best diet and to eat the foods that are optimal for you, as it is

Compare Popular Diet's [to the Base Functional Diet]

In their best form, all the diets that are popular at the moment, including Atkins, are diets that focus on real foods: lots of fruits and vegetables, good-quality protein sources, and healthy fats. There are also different views on the logic behind each diet, as well as its applications. My best diet would be one that would help those who want to be healthy and fit by

On the Paleo Diet, the main goal is to have a diet based on the most natural, well-adapted foods. This diet should be based on foods our ancestors ate. It should allow whole grains, dairy, beans, and nuts to be eaten at will. The base function diet focuses on eliminating allergens and inflammatory foods.

This program is a way to give people who are interested in healthier eating a chance to modify their nutritional habits. It uses the basic information of a base functional diet but does not allow any sweet foods or desserts such as honey.

A low-carb diet can be a quick way to lose weight by restricting carbohydrates. This diet is a combination of fat-free foods such as cheese, meat, yogurt or cottage cheese, and non-caloric sweeteners as long as they do not breach the set caloric or carbohydrate levels. A "celebration food" is scheduled in at the end to show that you are losing weight. Instead of following a low-carb diet, a high-protein

Mediterranean diet. Like the basic nutrition diet, a Mediterranean Diet emphasizes whole real foods. Whole grains and legumes are emphasized while fats are discouraged. Fish is a priority as seafood, and poultry is a top source of protein, while red meats are discouraged.

Detoxification. This means to rid the body of undesirable substances and toxins which can cause illness and mortality. Many people believe that a detox diet and cleanse is effective because the body is adept at detoxifying itself. A healthy diet, however, prevents ill effects through the body's natural ability to excrete toxins from the body. Detoxification diets may help boost the immune system and improve general health, but they can also cause severe harm to the body

6 A DIET DEDICATED TO ATHLETES

DASH (Dietary Approaches to Stop Hypertension) (high blood pressure) diet discourages people from eating processed foods in favor of fruits and vegetables. As well, DASH encourages people to consume more lean meat, nuts, and whole grains.

Consistent vegetarians. These eat primarily vegetables, fruits, grains, seeds, beans, nuts, and seeds. They may also consume some dairy and eggs. Sometimes, they do not eat meat, fish, or poultry. They avoid most processed foods and refined grains, including white flour products, candy, and soft drinks.

Many foods retain most of their vitamins when they are eaten raw, but others retain more nutrition when cooked. It is healthy to eat both raw and cooked foods.

The elimination diet is similar but not the same as the base functional diet because with it, much attention is paid to inflammatory foods such as sugar and processed food such as white sugar and processed grains such as white rice.

Too many diets force all of the foods out of your diet at the same time. When you do this, you don't know exactly why the change is working because there are too many different types of foods you have been consuming.

Chapter Two

THE PROBLEM OF FOOD INTOLERANCE

Although food is used for many purposes, it can be misused to maintain our daily lifestyle or to compete in our social relationships. When eating, people can choose the right foods for good health, or they can choose to eat the wrong foods to get a competitive edge.

A healthy diet is especially important for athletes because consuming the wrong foods can lead to inflammation that hinders healing. If your body has to constantly fight inflammation, you will perform and recover poorly. Eating the right foods will allow you to get better and recover faster. Athletes should eat the right foods to improve performance and mental clarity and reduce the risk of injury. In endurance sports, you may have to eat special diets; think about what you will need to achieve your goals and make the right decisions if you plan to go for marathons, Ironmans, and the like.

Where THE PROBLEM ENDS

8   A DIET DEDICATED TO ATHLETES
WHY

Food is a complex set of nutrients that are needed to fuel your body. Food provides energy, and also helps you to digest, absorb, and utilize the energy in the foods that you eat. Energy fuels the muscles and also provides your brain with energy. It is important to eat a balanced, nutritious diet in order to have a healthy body and mind.

A human's gastrointestinal tract is part of his or her digestive system. Although it is not the most obvious organ, it has many interactions with other parts of the body and plays a role in maintaining human health and function. It is very important to grasp because if an individual does not tolerate a particular food, the reaction to it can range anywhere in the body, from the skin to the brain, and can produce serious problems. For example, skin reactions, headaches, and trouble focusing are symptoms which may indicate food intolerances, such as gluten or dairy in gluten-free foods, soy, or lactose in lactose-free foods.

The gastrointestinal tract is the body's main barrier to harmful molecules. Every day, people ingest a variety of beneficial compounds and bacteria. Many of these molecules are needed for health and well-being and others can be harmful. The gut wall, which is just a thin sheet of cells, selectively lets both beneficial nutrients and toxic molecules into the body and blocks out harmful ones.

Leaky gut or gut barrier failure is a condition in which the gut barrier gets too tight, or too weak. When the gut barrier is too tight, the small molecules, such as food or bacteria, are too small to pass through the gut. This causes food to enter the blood stream. Bacteria and other toxins can also pass through this barrier. When the gut barrier gets too weak, it permeabilizes and lets in substances that usually shouldn't pass through.

Chapter Three

How healthy is your gut?

Many people don't realize that less than 10 percent of our own cells actually are us. The majority are bacteria that live in our intestine, and most of these bacteria reside in the intestines.

Your gut is a complex ecosystem of microorganisms that helps manage your body's health. The health of the wall that surrounds the intestine affects your immune system. In fact, your intestines are the front line of defense for your immune system. When you nurture them and keep them healthy by eating a nutritious diet, they will take care of you in return.

Only in recent years has the understanding of the millions of bacteria within our guts advanced, and with it, our burgeoning understanding of how this microbial community governs so many aspects of our health. The research into the microbes in our gut is just starting to get in its stride. We are just starting to get a glimpse of how various types of species of microbes first inhabit and then flourish in our guts, how much

12   A DIET DEDICATED TO ATHLETES

variation there is in the types and amounts of microbes among individuals, and how these communities reflect or determine aspects of health that may seem unrelated. Already it has been recognized that gut bacteria are important, along with other factors (such as diet, stress, and immune system function), to the risk of cardiovascular disease, musculoskeletal disease, bowel disorders, Crohn's disease, colon cancer, depression, and non-alcoholic fatty liver disease. People who suffer from these conditions have different varieties of gut bacteria,

High-performance athletes have a less than healthy food intake - which affects their metabolic function. They must also monitor their use of antibiotics because this too negatively affects their gut flora.

Poor diet affects each person differently. For example, obese people can't tolerate the usual foods people eat. Many people find foods like white bread, pasta, and sweets to be fattening and don't enjoy them. Conversely, others are able to maintain their weight on a good diet by eating many vegetables, brown rice, fish, and lean meats. It depends on the type of bacteria in the gut. People who have a healthy diet have bacteria in their gut that like to eat carbohydrates and protein, so that their body has no trouble absorbing the energy.

There are ongoing studies on the role of gut bacteria in treating conditions and diseases. In some cases, bacteria have been transplanted as a treatment for obesity. We have also seen successful fecal transplants in the treatment of certain illnesses. As farfetched as these ideas may seem, we are only beginning to consider the role probiotics and prebiotics play in good health.

Your bacteria are important, and you want to look after them.

What are probiotics and prebiotics?

What you are thinking about when you say probiotics is not really what probiotics are. You should know there are many types of probiotic bacteria. Probiotics are simply the good bacteria. Probiotic foods are live microorganisms that promote the growth of these healthy bacteria in the intestines. However, you should also eat the prebiotics, which are the fibers and other nutrients found in vegetables and fruits that help to grow the probiotic bacteria you consume. You should also take dietary probiotics as part of a healthy diet.

Chapter Four

UNDERSTANDING FOOD INTOLERANCES

The terms *allergy, intolerance*, and *sensitivity* are used interchangeably throughout the medical and nutrition world. However, it is important to be aware of the distinctions between each of these terms because they are not identical. For example, an allergy is a kind of sensitivity in which something (a food, a medicine, an insect bite) causes an immediate physical response that can be short-lived and sometimes even fatal. Intolerance is a difference in a reaction that cannot be identified as an allergy. Sensitivities are a feeling of discomfort or weakness that results in certain people from the ingestion of specific foods. In athletes, such as weight-lifters, this sensation can cause a feeling of lethargy, weakness, and loss of concentration.

You can trust your gut when you are hungry and full, upset or fine. It's also important to take the time to discuss your diet

16   A DIET DEDICATED TO ATHLETES

with a nutritionist, who may be able to help you find the foods that suit your needs best.

It is important to distinguish food intolerance from allergies, which usually require the same medical attention and testing. However, food intolerances can have a bad effect on one's health. A lack of proper nutrition in the short term can lead to a decline in immune system function, while having an immune system that is compromised can lead to frequent infections and other health problems.

ALLERGIES *vs.* INTOLERANCE

The most serious consequences of food allergies are asthma and anaphylactic shock. They are more common than many people realize. People who are allergic to nuts, milk, seafood, and egg are most susceptible. Symptoms of a mild allergy may appear within minutes of exposure. For example, a child who is allergic to peanuts might experience hives, watery eyes, and itching. Anaphylactic shock, which can be fatal, may occur from

The causes of allergies include insufficiency of specific substances necessary for the immune system to function normally; imbalance of the immune system and its response; an overactive immune system that produces antibodies when the body does not need them; and underactive or absent immune system.14 In general, allergic reactions occur immediately or within several hours of ingesting the substance or food in question and then dissipate within about half an hour. Although allergic reactions are usually mild, they can be life-threatening.15

Gastrointestinal problems are not always caused by food or dietary issues. For the majority of people who aren't experiencing an allergy, it is more difficult to discern between a food intolerance and a real disease. In this situation, people assume that it's a food intolerance rather than a real problem. For example, a person may not recognize a connection between a food intolerance and skin problems. We will learn more about this connection in the Skin chapter.

Cravings can be an indicator of the need to avoid foods which aggravate the hormonal system. A craving for a food or drink can be a signal that your body is addicted to the hormones histamine and cortisol which are released when you consume such foods. The craving may last for a good while after the offending food or beverage is consumed even if you have consumed just a little.

Some foods that have been identified as mood-boosting are not that great for you. As a result of diet restrictions, some of us start to feel worse than when we were eating junkier fare. Removing these "feel-good" foods from our diet may help with

18   A DIET DEDICATED TO ATHLETES

this anxiety. The good news is that if you are truly able to avoid these foods, you will feel much better.

Foods can contribute to food and environmental sensitivity. The amount of a particular chemical you may become sensitive to is a threshold, which may not have a noticeable effect on your health until you accumulate a high concentration of that chemical over time.

Eating habits 2. The best diet to follow Paraphrase: The best diet 3. When you stop Paraphrase: When you

These are just some of the many reasons why we have different foods sensitivities — some genetic. Some of my readers may have a genetic sensitivity that they are not aware of, but could change their habits and feel better. It can be really upsetting to know that you might have a problem, especially if you feel that you have no control over what you eat, that you are a weak and helpless person, and that your partner or family don't understand you. There is hope. You can make changes and get better.

Although the scope of this book does not include all the factors that can cause, contribute to or confound food intolerances, it is important to understand how complex our bodies are and how difficult it can be to decipher the cause of our symptoms.

Children can grow out of food allergies or intolerances at any age. But, when the allergy or intolerance is introduced by a parasite or is from a severe illness, such as pneumonia, it may be harder to diagnose. Food intolerance can also occur during or after pregnancy. A combination of lifestyle factors, genetics, and hormonal changes in the body can contribute to food intolerances, such as lactose intolerance.

How external forces *can exacerbate or cause intolerance*

The strong connection between the gut and mind plays an important role in the presentation and severity of digestive symptoms. With regards to stress reduction and other lifestyle factors, the role of diet can be assessed.

Alcohol can increase gut wall permeability. The effect can be increased when combined with other irritants, such a caffeine.

weakened immunity. Because the gut is the central control point for the body's immune defenses, any time the immune system is under siege by illness, its ability to cope with digestion and maintenance of the gut barrier may be compromised.

Hygiene. Hygiene is a way to keep a house clean and healthy. When it is too clean, our body cannot function well.

Vitamin D. New research has revealed that **vitamin D** may play an important role in how the immune system functions and the health of the cells in the gut. This is why **low vitamin D levels** are associated with a wide range of conditions and

20   A DIET DEDICATED TO ATHLETES

The kinds of bacteria in our gut will change depending on the food we eat and the use of antibiotics. As the bacteria in our organs evolve, it can affect how well our organs work and potentially cause new diseases.

Parasites. Physical damage and changes in gut bacteria can also be a danger when parasites are not treated and managed properly. This is something to be managed with a medical professional.

When learning to cook, it can be hard to know which ingredients might cause a reaction. To figure that out, it's important to learn about the causes of food sensitivities.

WHY

In most cases, people don't realize their food allergies are causing their problems. In some cases, the connection between food allergies and more serious conditions, such as skin ailments, may be missed or misunderstood. It's rare for someone to have a single food allergy, but sometimes two or more different allergies may exist. When someone experiences a new allergy, it can be difficult to find the actual problem food. Symptoms may go unnoticed because they are a normal occurrence for the person, or they may overlap with other conditions, such as an inflammatory bowel syndrome.

Some people believe that certain foods or food groups cause intolerance. For instance, a person might believe dairy causes intolerance. However, the person likely is intolerant to gluten. For this person, if dairy is eliminated, the intestinal damage from the lactase enzyme may not be completely fixed. Even if the person has a gluten-free diet, the intestinal damage that resulted in intolerance to dairy is likely still in place. Other people may suffer from lactose intolerance even if they don't have gluten intolerance.

We are often scared of the unknown. We may not be sure if a food intolerance is affecting our health. It is helpful to gather information from others who have had similar experiences to yours. For example, you could ask your mother if she has noticed your symptoms as you have described them and also listen to how she coped when she had to change her diet. You could ask a friend with a similar problem how he or she coped. You could also get a nutritionist's opinion about whether you are eating correctly. Finally, you can ask your parents to support you when you decide to change your diet.

WHY FOOD INTOLERANCES ARE UP

Studies show that food allergies and intolerances are increasing across the globe. People without a medical diagnosis of food allergies and intolerances often self-diagnose them themselves. They do not receive adequate treatment for their medical condition, and food allergy and intolerance rates are under-reported by as much as 40%.[21]

22 A DIET DEDICATED TO ATHLETES

The prevalence of celiac disease has increased at a rapid rate. Currently, the Centers for Disease Control estimates that there are over 3.5 million Americans with celiac disease. The disease is known to be genetically related to type 1 and type 2 diabetes, obesity and osteoporosis. Researchers discovered a high rate of celiac disease in many of these diseases. This suggests that environmental changes may have triggered, or exacerbated, the disease.

It's no surprise that more people are being diagnosed with celiac disease than in years past. Because people prefer the more modern style of bread, in combination with gluten-filled foods like pizza and pasta, it's likely that we are eating more gluten than past generations were. We are also seeing an increase in gluten sensitivity, though many people may not even know about it.

Our food sources have changed dramatically over time. We now have less variety in our diets. The foods that are available are mostly derived from wheat, corn, and dairy products. These components contain gluten and casein, which can lead to inflammation and cause intolerances.

Even as it increases its dependence on nonrenewable resources, the United States faces an additional problem due to the growing number of environmentally-sensitive foods.

The question of whether food sensitivities are increasing may be too difficult to ascertain.

Chapter Five

Athlete's or food intolerance

Eating gluten-free, eliminating dairy, and going on a special diet are common among athletes. And some of them do it to improve their performance. They might go on a special diet for a short period of time, such as to make their race weight, or maybe they are trying to improve their health. Many athletes think the benefits of being healthy far outweigh the disadvantages of having to eat a particular diet.

Because the health of an Olympic competitor can be vital, it is worth the time and effort to identify and eliminate hidden nutrition issues. Whether they are associated with food or medical allergies, nutrition is often overlooked by athletes in training and competition, so it's worth exploring.

Many athletes are able to detect problems in their performance or their body's response to the work they are doing. This heightened sense of awareness may be responsible for athletes recognizing their dietary choices are

26   A DIET DEDICATED TO ATHLETES

impacting their ability to perform at the highest level. Sports may also prompt athletes to seek out a cause for their symptoms.

Furthermore, the increased permeability of the gut may lead to food intolerance. The immune system may be activated whenever there is a change in the environment of the gut. Physical stress, the activity of exercise, and the dietary intake of the subject all can alter the gut's environment.

The physical symptoms that result from exercise may resemble those of a food intolerance. However, exercise doesn't trigger this disorder. Instead, a combination of low glycogen stores (fueling) and high volume training can lead to intolerance symptoms. When these factors are present during an intense training session, they may cause discomfort and even GI distress.

STRESS

Whether they are engaged during training, or they prepare for a test or performance, athletes are always experiencing stress. Their gastrointestinal systems are particularly affected by the stress, whether physical, mental or emotional.

This may include a lack of sleep, fatigue, stress, pain, poor nutrition, illness, injury, family, and mental issues.

The stresses of professional sports and exercise can disrupt the intestinal lining and make athletes more sensitive to certain foods. As a result, they may have more difficulty digesting certain foods. Therefore, it's crucial to understand these stresses when considering the impact of exercise on food tolerance in athletes.

Regular exercise leads to immunity levels that are enhanced in general. In healthy athletes, immune defense systems are temporarily depressed in the hours following an intense workout. Regular training exercises can lead to more food intolerances. Training can also increase stress on the body, which may decrease the body's immune response to food intolerances.

MECHANICAL FACTORS

Many health problems, such as intestinal ills, can be traced to the food we eat. When your body is stressed, as can be during exercise, blood flow to your intestinal tract diminishes, which leads to the increased passage of food particles into the bloodstream. The result is food intolerance and the possible occurrence of symptoms that you don't have when you aren't exercising. For instance, you may become sensitive to foods containing gluten. You might also experience headaches, stomach pain, and dizziness.

28   A DIET DEDICATED TO ATHLETES

A sudden bout of extreme stress may trigger lactose intolerance. Or, the body's inflammatory response may be affected by the exercise itself, creating GI upsets with food.

The physical movements during exercise, such as running or cycling, cause more reflux episodes than sitting on a bike or bench at rest. However, the jarring effects of running may also cause an imbalance in the intestines, which can result in food intolerances. The same logic that applies to stationary exercise can be applied to more sedentary tasks: sitting at a desk or slumping on a couch can also prevent the GI tract from functioning as desired.

NUTRITION BODY FITNESS & STRENGTH FITNESS FITNESS & FITNESS

Because the bacteria in your gut are influenced by diet, exercise, illness, antibiotics, and stress, athletes must be mindful of their health and habits when choosing foods and training their bodies.

Sports foods that consist of a lot of sugar alter gut bacteria and reduce their ability to protect the gut wall. Athletes who eat a diet comprised of a lot of sugar experience changes in the gut that impair their ability to keep intestines in a healthy state.

Refined high-energy foods: Athletes like pasta noodles, couscous, cereals, bagels, and bread. Foods with high carbohydrates provide an energy boost, but they are lower in nutritional density. If athletes rely too heavily on these types of foods, they lack nutrients that are high in quality.

Celiac disease is an autoimmune disease characterized by damage to the intestinal lining due to the intolerance of gluten. Athletes with celiac disease avoid wheat and other gluten-containing foods to prevent diarrhea and other intestinal disturbances. In the absence of intestinal problems, some athletes may still experience symptoms that cause them to avoid gluten for other reasons. Eating clean and being aware of gluten ingestion may help prevent or relieve these symptoms.

Anti-inflammatories. You have trained hard to reach your goals, and paid your entry fees, booked travel and accommodations, and informed all your friends and relatives of your plans. Now, you are faced with a serious injury. Perhaps you pushed too far and were just clumsy. This could happen to anyone. If this happens, you won't be able to back out.

Your starting spot in sports is so important and losing it is embarrassing. It puts a bad taste in everyone's mouth and is a shame to the team. When this happens, anti-inflammatories are your best friend. They can help you be active and still be able to compete. But, the wrong drugs can cause long-term

30 A DIET DEDICATED TO ATHLETES

damage to your gut lining and raise the risk of a serious infection like a UTI.

The human body becomes exhausted from hard or intense physical activity that stimulates the immune system. The frequency and severity of illnesses for athletes is high because they are not fully rested at the beginning of the season. Some athletes take antibiotics in an attempt to prevent infections. It's important to understand that antibiotics do not relieve infections by killing viruses.

Chapter Six

When you want to perform well, eat well.

The demands of professional sports may lead to food intolerance, which can sometimes be a side effect of the demands of playing or training for an athletic event. Many athletes are aware of the problem from playing at unhealthy levels, or through feeling sluggish or tired on a daily basis, but maybe they don't see other possible connections. We'll tell you how common this problem is for athletes, and how to recognize it and cure it.

GI ISSUES

I have found that all runners suffer from some sort of gastrointestinal condition before, during, and after a run. It is normal and, at times, even enjoyable to have gastronomical issues in running. This is a healthy way of getting rid of some stress and, moreover, I enjoy it. In my opinion, it is as normal as having chest pains and coughing fits before running.

32   A DIET DEDICATED TO ATHLETES

Most exercise-induced GI distress may be prevented with proper fluid intake, eating light and healthy snacks, and/or keeping a supply of antacids at hand. There are several types of GI distress. Stomach cramps are usually the result of stomach acid backing up in the small intestine. Running to the bathroom to pass a bowel movement is actually the body's way of flushing out this extra acid that might have built up. The rectum may also get irritated, causing a painful flush.

Many people have gastritis, which may cause stomach pain, vomiting, stomach bloating, burping, and nausea. In addition, some people have acute upper digestive problems such as peptic ulcer disease, which causes severe stomach cramps accompanied by pain and intense, sharp feeling.

The body's digestive system, which includes the stomach and intestines, is responsible for storing and digesting food. When digestive function is adequate, food is transformed into energy that is essential to a muscle-building workout or an endurance event. GI problems can be caused by excessive or insufficient use of the digestive system, a food intolerant response, a dietary pattern that contributes to the problem, or stress related to the event. If you feel gastrointestinal issues that persist, it may be time to seek medical advice.

Most sports foods contain fructose. Since that sugar can be difficult to handle, some athletes have managed to avoid

WHEN YOU WANT TO PERFORM WELL, EAT WELL.   33

having it when they're running or competing and, for others, the sugar can cause a true intolerance.

While baking might be delicious, the exercise may not. However, exercising early before eating a high carbohydrate meal may prevent you from overeating. For example, if you eat too much food, you may be able to better tolerate the exercise.

GI issues are usually manageable if you follow a sensible diet and schedule when eating and exercising in your long run. They can also be reversed by avoiding sensitive foods and improving your hydration. When they are ignored or severe, they can lead to complications like blood loss in the stool, which are difficult to heal. These issues can require medical intervention.

How *to troubleshoot* your

The following are some reasons why a diet may fail.

FODMAPs. The sensitivity to certain carbohydrates can be increased above threshold tolerance levels due to the fact that the levels of anxiety or stress associated with an event is increased. People who are sensitive to FODMAPs should try to stay away from food that contain FODMAPs for 24–48 hours prior to

34   A DIET DEDICATED TO ATHLETES

Fructose. This common ingredient is one of the Fermentation Odor Material that can cause gi problems for athletes. If the foods that you're fueling with contains Fructose, pay close attention to whether malabsorption or intolerance can be to blame.

Lactose. This is often a transient intolerance that only presents during exercise. To minimize GI distress in such cases, consume dairy products in the morning, lunch, and dinner, and only do so in small amounts.

In a study, athletes were asked if they needed to consume caffeine on a daily basis in order to maintain their athletic performance. Some of them stated that they can't even tolerate caffeine before workouts, so they need to avoid it before their workouts.

Other *food intolerances*.

What to eat before working out. Eating food prior to working out usually increases the amount of liquid which is absorbed into the body. While eating before exercising causes no problem for most people, some individuals have an increase in blood volume which may lead to lightheadedness and/or

It might be wise to limit your daily intake of fat or fiber. This can make things move too quickly in your GI tract which could be uncomfortable.

WHEN YOU WANT TO PERFORM WELL, EAT WELL. 35

Sports drinks, gels, bars, or other foods that have too much carbohydrate may impair the gastric emptying process and reduce intestinal fluid absorption.

Dehydration makes stomach acid more likely to come out in your stomach, and it can slow the emptying of the stomach after a meal. When athletes drink enough water to satisfy thirst, they are able to lose weight during workouts. In races that take place in hot weather, athletes need to drink enough to avoid dehydration.

Injuries are caused by race-day situations

Stress and anxiety can be controlled with **preparation**, **chatting with family**, **listening to music**,

NSAIDs and **antibiotics** both increase intestinal permeability. These can cause intestinal issues without the existence of an intolerance.

Some sports like cycling can put pressure on the abdomen, possibly leading to upper gastrointestinal tract. In cycling, some bike fit can reduce this discomfort. For example, in other sports, the balancing act between optimizing posture for gastrointestinal comfort versus performance can tip into or out of any way, depend on the level of the athlete and the demands of the race.

36   A DIET DEDICATED TO ATHLETES

Vibration of the Gut: When you exercise, such as running or practicing sports to perform gymnastic moves, friction and irritation of the gut can cause diarrhea or stomach pain. You can also experience diarrhea or stomach pain after consuming irritating foods or not staying hydrated. The solution, however, is to minimize the effects of friction. Do the following: practice appropriate fueling; avoid irritating

It could be that the food allergy or intolerance is being affected by your training.

BODY COMPOSITION

Body weight determines the capacity to perform, which is why athletes compete with a preference for those with lower body weights. But this has many negative health implications if the athlete overeats, even on a controlled diet, or is inactive. Athletes must take care to stay lean, but sometimes this means gaining body fat to provide more muscle mass and strength, but not body weight.

Many people have the goal of losing weight, but diet quality may be just as important as calories. When a person is trying to lose weight, the best thing he or she can do is stop eating processed foods, refined carbs, and sugars. Eating a raw-food diet may be an effective strategy to lose weight as it decreases the chances of inflammation from hidden food intolerances.

WHEN YOU WANT TO PERFORM WELL, EAT WELL. 37

Food intolerances can contribute to weight gain in several ways:

Eating certain kinds of foods, like certain foods, can set off a cycle of cravings. These cravings can be strong and difficult to overcome.

Inflammation. Swelling is common when inflammation results from food intolerance. Bloating or puffiness can be reduced by eliminating or avoiding problem foods. [1]: http://www.

Mood swings. The sudden changes in mood are often caused by food intolerances. An emotionally sensitive person often finds food and eating experiences to help soothe their moods. This, in turn, contributes to weight gain.

The idea of losing weight doesn't work for many people, and athletes can be affected by the same problem. Instead of trying to deprive yourself of calories, what if you looked at other options like taking advantage of vitamin D and using high-carbohydrate drinks that contain calcium?

Some bodybuilders need to put on muscle and increase their weight when training heavily or to meet the demands of training to build size and strength. This usually means that they are not eating well for the majority of their training cycle. Because intestinal enzymes and the ability to absorb nutrients are hindered by food intolerances, they may be experiencing

38   A DIET DEDICATED TO ATHLETES

mild food allergies and nutrient deficiencies. This may lead to problems in gaining weight and building muscle mass.

ILLNESS & INJURY

Athletes, and elite athletes in particular, are known for always being on the brink of illness and/or injury. Much of this has to do with chronic stress, both the mechanical stress on muscles, bones, joints, and ligaments that disposes us to injury and the physical and emotional stress related to hard training. Chronic stress can leave a healthy athlete in a run-down state with low-grade chronic inflammation because the body's immune system is perpetually fighting off infection. Inflammation is also present with injuries. You know that red-hot throbbing and swelling you experience after you twist an ankle? That's inflammation—the body's natural protective response to injury—which is extremely beneficial in the short term. But prolonged inflammation is not such great news.

A food intolerance can make it difficult to heal an injury or an illness where inflammation is present. For example, a food intolerance may make it difficult for the digestive system to heal after surgery. A gluten intolerance may make it difficult to heal an injury where the muscles are sore.

When illness or injury strike, it is helpful to reduce the inflammation in the body. By eating a diet that is rich in fruits, vegetables, and whole grains, you can reduce the rate

WHEN YOU WANT TO PERFORM WELL, EAT WELL. 39

of illness and injury while promoting a healthier body. Foods you can eat include avocados, apples, bananas, beans, berries, carrots, celery, corn, cucumbers, green leafy vegetables, garlic, lemons, limes, onions, oranges, pears, peppers, spinach, strawberries, and tomatoes.

On the other hand, illness can also precipitate a food intolerance. It is like a person's immune system can be suppressed by stress, so that they can be sensitive to foods that previously didn't bother them.

RECOVERY & SLEEP

Good sleep is so important for our physical and mental health that a lack of it is comparable to torture. This is shown in studies about how sleep deprivation is one of the worst forms of torture we could be subjected to. Parents, teachers, and others with child-care responsibilities have complained about their own lack of sleep and have lost weight due to sleep deprivation. The most effective way to increase sleep is to follow certain diet and lifestyle practices.

These sleep patterns are affected by the foods we eat. Reactions to caffeine, alcohol, and some foods, including large or spicy meals or alcohol, may hinder sleep quality. The chemical reactions to certain foods can account for the sleep problems associated with them. Gluten is considered the most problematic.

40   A DIET DEDICATED TO ATHLETES

If you are having trouble sleeping because of diet, consider your diet's impact on your sleep. For example, could it be that you overeat or drink too much, or are you stressed out?

COGNITIVE EFFECTS

In addition to the physical qualifications of team sports, including speed, agility, and strength, cognition plays a crucial role in athletic performance (as it does in all other aspects of life). Reflex actions, hand-eye coordination, as well as tactical ability are crucial elements for athletes and those who participate in endurance events. Some sports are timed to the millisecond, such as a marathon where athletes are separated only through electronic photo finishes. Other events are played out over countless hours and physical and mental stress

To be mentally alert and strong is vital for an outstanding racing performance. Knowing how to think clearly and quickly, and how to define a situation in a positive framework, are important tools you need in safe racing.

It's often said that if you can influence your attitude, then you can easily influence your success. So people often alter their diet in order to influence their attitude.

While it's important to follow a fitness plan before a major competition, it is more important to continue to develop your body. Consistently training your body to achieve fitness goals

WHEN YOU WANT TO PERFORM WELL, EAT WELL. 41

may be more effective than competing in a big event when you are mentally or physically drained. Original: A positive attitude and the dogged determination to succeed that is what sets athletes apart is what sets the most high-ranking officials in sports apart.

GENDER & HORMONES

There are many differences between women and men (not only in body size, but also in eating habits and tolerance to food products). This, in turn, affects the body type of the "gender-fluid."

Most women have more food intolerances and allergies than do their male counterparts. The cause is unclear. However, a hormone imbalance may be involved. Women who experience menstrual cycles may need to be more aware of what they eat and how it affects them in different phases of their monthly cycles.

"The female athlete triad comprises a series of health issues that occur especially in women involved in endurance sports. It should be distinguished from athletic amenorrhea, or irregular periods, and low energy availability, or amenorrhea. The triad is associated with low energy intake and abnormal hormone levels such as a low level of estrogen and luteinizing hormone, as well as an inability to make and maintain an ideal weight."

42   A DIET DEDICATED TO ATHLETES

A low-energy diet can affect a woman's hormonal balance, which can decrease her bone density and result in menstrual irregularities or even lead to the development of a condition known as female athlete triad. Due to the loss of estrogen, low-energy diet can lead to the development of stress fractures in the bone. If a female athlete is sidelined with a stress fracture, it may not be until later that her illness is diagnosed and treated. In some cases, her menstrual periods may not be regular. Low-energy diets can help female athletes gain energy and performance. But if the diet does not provide enough calories to meet the woman's energy needs, her hormone levels can decrease, which can contribute to bone loss.

Reproductive function is affected by both energy intake and expenditure. Both caloric and carbohydrate intake are important to maintaining healthy hormone function.

The gut has hormone receptors in different parts along it, and is a distinct and important link to the endocrine system. Even though we don't have a complete understanding of these links, we do know that the gut can directly affect endocrine function.

One cause for infertility or pregnancy complications may involve poor food intake. For example, celiac and gluten intolerance may impair nutrient absorption. In fact, nutritional

WHEN YOU WANT TO PERFORM WELL, EAT WELL. 43

deficiencies have been linked to infertility and/or pregnancy complications.

Women and men who aren't trying to conceive, whether in the near future or ever, should still want to make sure that their bodies are in good shape. They shouldn't change hormone levels.

COMMIT to finding the best foods

I will start to figure out what my best foods are by improving the way I eat and take care of my body. By knowing how to nourish my body properly, it will be easier to build muscle and lose weight, and I will enjoy more energy and vitality.

Chapter Seven

FIXING YOUR DIET

People need to eat food in different ways. One person might eat diet food for breakfast and eat a homecooked meal at night, while others might eat the same diet food at night and eat a homecooked meal at breakfast.

There are three things that you must do to get started with your diet. These steps can help you in selecting the foods that are good for you, and they will lead you to your fitness goal.

It is important to eliminate foods that are bad for our health and impede our performance. Some foods have a strong impact on the body. For example, some people have difficulty digesting dairy products. These foods can be detrimental because they change our health and may increase our risk of certain diseases, such as diabetes.

As new evidence has emerged, chronic inflammation has become recognized as the root for many health conditions as well as diseases.

46   A DIET DEDICATED TO ATHLETES

If inflammation becomes chronic, it may be more serious than an injury or bacterial infection. In the following paragraphs, information may be found about foods that are known to increase inflammation and those that help keep it in check.

Whether in competition, in a work-out, or on the run, carbohydrates should be used efficiently in our diets and should be combined with other types of food when appropriate. These foods can cause inflammation, which slows the body's recovery. But there are a few foods that are best avoided altogether.

Eliminate or minimize the specific foods that could possibly be causing intolerance symptoms. The second category of food intolerances are highly individual. The individualized elimination diet is often needed in order to determine the foods they are intolerant to. Some intolerances may be mild and can be controlled with a trial of an elimination diet. Others may require the patient to follow a strict diet that requires elimination of all trigger foods. Some foods are less common culprits than others. Fructose is often responsible for bloating and gas among many people. Fructose, however, is often consumed with other foods. This fact makes the elimination diet even more critical. Fructose is often found in such foods as sugar-free jellies and soft drinks.

The final phase of the process is to **identify what you can have foods that are well tolerated, and reintroduce more of those foods.** Your food diary will help you identify all intolerances and identify what you can have. Variety is important because it is healthy for you and you enjoy food in the long term.

Don't eat the unhealthy foods that cause inflammation

Not all foods are created equal. Certain foods carry more risks than others. Some foods should be eliminated from regular diets while healthy diets should include foods that carry less risk. The foods above pose more health risks than healthy options, so they should be eliminated from, or at least minimized in, your diet.

> Processed and packaged foods

> Refined grains

> Sugars and sweeteners

Hydrogenated oils, trans fats and some animal fats.

> Artificial colors and flavors

This food list might seem like a short list, but the reality is that most foods consumed in the Western world are composed of one or more of these types of food. The fact that most people consume food that includes these types of food is problematic. If you regularly eat some of these foods, it's possible that they'll

48   A DIET DEDICATED TO ATHLETES

have a negative impact on your heath. As with any habit, it's better to not consume

There's a shocking amount of nutrition-related food waste in your household. You spend more than 30 percent of your food budget on unhealthy processed foods and beverages that contribute to the US obesity epidemic. You spend more than 10 percent of your food budget each month on frozen and canned meals. About one in ten of the food you spend on fresh fruits and vegetables goes to waste instead of eating it.

Processed & packaged foods

If you were offered all the foods available to eat in the world, you would recognize that the options are small. In the U.S. market alone, there are about 20,00 new foods introduced into supermarkets every year. About 25 percent are confectionaries or snack foods, while a further 20 percent are under the beverage category. This variation in food choices is not because we have too many choices in the grocery store. Instead, the variety of foods we eat is relatively homogeneous. And even though we encounter many options, and even a variety of foods in the grocery store, our options are surprisingly limited and they are fairly similar. To

Foods made of corn, soy, wheat or a derivative of one are widely used in everyday processed food, even one a bite at a time, such as breakfast cereals. Almost 40 percent of the calories consumed in the U.S. come from these food sources. The best way to avoid them is to eat only whole foods like vegetables, fruits, and lean meats.

The average American consumes roughly 150 pounds of sugar annually, and this number has been rising. 52

REFINED GRAINS

The rise of food allergies, celiac disease and other food intolerances may be linked to how wheat is produced, prepared, packaged, and brought to market. In a way, processed wheat products have become the same as the processed foods we already recognize and eat — they're not as varied and offer less variety in variety and quality. This is why the average American eats more refined products than fresh produce.

Refined carbohydrate foods, such as white flour and pasta, are converted to sugar within the person's bloodstream. This conversion of blood sugar (glucose) to fuel occurs in the liver and muscles. When this conversion of blood sugar to fuel exceeds glucose demand, blood sugar levels increase. When the body has excess insulin, more sugar is pulled from stores for conversion to energy and this can increase inflammation levels. When a person has an energy deficit, they are in danger of becoming hypoglycemic and experiencing glucose deficiency.

50   A DIET DEDICATED TO ATHLETES

It's important to give your body the nutrition it needs, even if it is only during intense physical exercise. Athletes at a certain level of their training routine may benefit from a carb-heavy diet, but nutritionists are also increasingly emphasizing the importance of a healthy diet for the general public with no specific athletic endeavors.

SUGARS & SWEETENERS

While it's true that athletes may be healthier than the population in general, it's also true that highly refined and processed carbs and sugars are still a significant part of their diets, whether in the form of specialized sports foods (e.g., drinks, bars, chews, gels), or even a justified reward following a hard workout with a cookie or ice cream. But a quick ice cream or cookie, after a workout, is not going to make someone healthier, regardless of how many calories they consume. In fact, they may be undermining their health by increasing their sugar intake.

Certain foods can act as drugs and trigger addictive responses in people with certain gut hormones. Some people actually become addicted to sugar, and others binge eat when they just have a taste. Since our ancestors needed to be able to track the availability of food and stock up when they were in short supply, we were naturally inclined to eat more of these foods.

However, it's not healthy to eat these foods in excess. Instead, we should try to reduce or eliminate them from our diets.

Spotting SUGAR

The word "ose" at the beginning of each of the words sugars below, except fructose. This project was created in class using the website,

Syrups and sweeteners.

-itol Usually denote a sugar alcohol and might be calorie-free, but there are some concerns related to these sweeteners that need to be researched so that the final decision can be made which one is the best.

Regular consumption of sugar can alter your blood sugar levels by the thousands. But artificial sweeteners can do even more harm to your health. The lining of your gastrointestinal tract can be damaged by artificial sweeteners, which can change the composition and numbers of your gut microbiota and reduce your immunity level. In the long run, eating a diet full of artificial sweeteners can affect your health and performance in every aspect of your lifestyle.

GOOD FATS

The ratio of omega-6 to omega-3 fats in the average diet is overwhelmingly skewed toward the more pro-inflammatory omega-6s, so it is important to get your omega-6s from the

52   A DIET DEDICATED TO ATHLETES

most healthful sources. Vegetables, fruit, nuts, and fish are all great sources of omega 3 fats, and it is best to eat them frequently.

If we consume foods that are not good for us, our bodies suffer. As humans we have been eating too many processed and artificial foods, and even our cows are not immune to it.

ARTIFICIAL

Anytime you see artificial color or flavor in a list of ingredients. This can be an all-too-familiar red flag that anything is amiss — from the actual food to the way it looks, tastes, and even what was said on the label. These artificial colors and flavors may be the hidden culprit of nonallergic reactions and intolerances.

The inflammatory foods that are abundant in our diet include red meats, eggs, dairy, poultry, and sugary foods. Eating these foods as part of our diet contributes to the inflammatory state that exists in many people. Simply avoiding these foods in our diet may help us feel better.

FRESH PRODUCE

We have all been given some excellent advice about eating vegetables. Perhaps you are among the most committed to following the recommendations and consume the recommended servings every day. It is a good day when you do. But most people fall far short of these goals. Maybe you just didn't know you were eating them all this time... You should understand that vegetables are delicious and they are an excellent way to enjoy every meal.

Think of the whole produce department at the grocery store. All of those different colors represent a variety of antioxidants and flavonoids.

Today, humans are the main source of free radicals. The process is something that's normal and necessary, but what's abnormal is when those free radicals do more harm than good. Our bodies have a limited ability to neutralize free radicals, or so-called reactive radicals. So we use antioxidants to help balance the equation. Antioxidants are found in foods like berries, vegetables, whole grains, and oil seeds.

Antioxidants, the important nutrients in fruits and vegetables, can be found in copper, zinc, selenium, vitamin E, vitamin C, and flavonoids. It is known that flavonoids and phytochemicals present in fruits and vegetables are believed to have even stronger antioxidant effects.

Flavonoids, also known as flavonols, are responsible for the color of plants. Many plant foods are high in flavonols. Research has shown that a diet high in plant-based foods offers health benefits. But, we are still not sure what all the health benefits are. Many types of flavonoids have been found to offer health benefits, however, the evidence is not entirely

54   A DIET DEDICATED TO ATHLETES

clear. For example, some studies have indicated that taking antioxidant supplements does not offer any additional health benefits.

NUTS & SEEDS

Eating healthy foods such as almonds is an excellent health strategy. Nuts and seeds are loaded with nutrients, fiber, and healthy proteins, which all play an important role in overall wellness. It is also easy to eat them because they are portable.

FRESH FRUIT & VEGETABLES

We should consume animal foods because they contain good nutrition like iron, zinc, iodine, phosphorous, copper, potassium, essential fatty acids, and vitamins. Some of these are only found in meat and eggs, and these can help our bodies.

just

And red meats, particularly beef, lamb, deer, and bison, provide food supplies containing iron and B vitamins, such as b12.

A vegetarian diet may be healthier than a meat diet as it provides plenty of vitamins, vitamins, and minerals.

Fish and shellfish have their own claim to fame. They are a good source of essential fatty acids and vitamin D, along with iodine, potassium, and zinc.

FIXING YOUR DIET　55

> The flesh of liver, chicken, and beef are among the richest sources of vitamins. Poultry liver is more nutritious than beef liver. Liver is rich in B vitamins. Chicken liver is richer in iron than beef liver. Beef liver is richer in protein than chicken liver. Liver contains a lot of nutrients such as vitamins A and D.

> Eggs are a type of food that cannot be classified as something that everyone needs, but it is a food that is recommended for everyone to include in their daily diet. They contain all the essential amino-acids along with vitamins A, B

Food and lifestyle are very important for humans. They are also important for animals. If an animal is healthy and has lead a happy life, then their meat (and/or eggs) will be produced in high quality.

NATURAL FATS

A new meta-analysis of the evidence shows that *fat* is good for you, not bad. There is no benefit to reducing saturated fats or replacing them with unsaturated fats. Instead, focus on eating mostly *fat* instead of empty, sweet and processed carbohydrates. People can't reduce saturated fat intake to the point that they become deficient in omega-3 fatty acids and omega-6 fatty acids.

The good news is that omega-3s are available from natural sources like wild-caught fish and other fatty sea foods. The bad

56 A DIET DEDICATED TO ATHLETES

news is that many of us have problems with either producing or absorbing them.

Vegan & Vegetarian Diets

It has become a common belief that veggie diets may be healthy and also that it may be the best diet for the human body. But veggie diets shouldn't be confused as the only natural way of eating. To truly be healthy a vegetarian diet needs to be well balanced.

Many people decide to follow a vegan or vegetarian diet to benefit their own health. They believe that animal products increase their risk of chronic illness. However, when people eat meat responsibly they don't have to worry about getting sick. Scientists have reported that the quality of meats sold in supermarkets is often low; therefore, any meat you buy needs to be fresh and healthy.

Vegan diets contain more plant-related nutrients than animal-derived nutrients. Vegans should be aware of the foods that they choose, such that they get enough calcium, iron, zinc, vitamin A, vitamin B12, vitamin D, omega-3 fatty acids, and protein.

On the basis that they are mostly found in animal products, vegetarians need supplements to meet the levels of the nutrients they can't get from a vegetarian diet. Vegans who eat eggs and dairy will find it easier to meet nutritional targets than vegans who don't eat dairy and eggs.

CPSIA information can be obtained
at www.ICGtesting.com
Printed in the USA
LVHW061605200722
723979LV00011B/185